INNER BLOCKS
TO
LOSING WEIGHT

Why You Lose The Battle More Than The Weight!

SIDNEY J. COHEN, PH.D.

ISBN: 1-4392-6523-2
ISBN-13: 9781439265239

TABLE OF CONTENTS

* * *

Chapter 1
AN OVERVIEW

* * *

"Shed those pounds we guarantee it!"
"Become the thin you!"
"This is the diet for YOU!"
"Lose 20 pounds in 6 weeks!"

Dina, an overweight friend of mine, and I were recently sitting at lunch discussing weight-loss advertisements like those above. Suddenly Dina reached out, gripped my arm tightly, and exclaimed, "Sid, you have no idea how lucky you are! Your insides don't start churning when you read or hear hyped-up words like those headlines about losing weight!" Once the numbness in my arm disappeared, I acknowledged her statement to be true, and for two reasons. First, I knew from years of friendship how often Dina's insides did in fact churn at the mention of ads on the subject of losing weight and keeping it off. Second, I know I am very fortunate that my stomach hardly ever churns at the mention of this particular subject.

The reason I don't get agitated like Dina is because my weight has held consistent within a ten-pound height-appropriate range for most of my adult life. This is not meant to boast or imply there's been anything easy about my weight remaining steady over the years. I simply consider myself fortunate to have had the luxury of disregarding promotions of the weight-loss industry.

Haven't you been seduced or tempted at one time or another by effusive promises and scintillating photographs in an illusion-creating weight-loss ad? Serial dieters (like yourself?) are often lured by ads assuring a transformation into a slender "femme fatale" or a handsome "Adonis" of a guy. However, the fact of the matter is: no reported studies have concluded that any diet or exercise program can accomplish such a make-over with any consistency.

Even the diet promoters profiting from these programs apparently do not believe they are as effective as their advertisements boast. After all, if those companies were confident of the results, disclaimers would not be tucked in a distant corner of their ads, far from the willowy woman or muscular male in the before-and-after photo. No doubt you've seen those disclaimers, especially these two staples: "Individual results may vary" and "results not typical." Frankly, we could all assume that if these programs were as effective as promised, no such disclaimers would ever be included. Nor of course would the recidivism rate for people regaining lost weight be anywhere as high as the generally accepted, quite disturbing estimate of over 90 percent!

Ninety-Seven Million American Adults are Overweight

Can you possibly estimate how many Joes and Josephines, desperate to lose weight, are out there dieting this very day? Although the rate of growth has slowed somewhat, the National Center for Health Statistics still reports that 34 percent of American adults are obese. In hard numbers, that totals seventy-two million people. The number jumps to ninety-seven million, the American Dietetic Association reports, when it includes American adults who are both overweight and obese.

The terms "obese" and "overweight" both refer to an excess of body fat. Frequently used interchangeably, they have distinct meanings, as determined by the level of a person's excess weight. Perhaps you have heard of a measurement of obesity created by health experts that uses a mathematical formula known as Body-Mass Index (BMI). A BMI greater than twenty-five is considered overweight and above thirty is considered obese. Current data from the Center for Disease Control and Prevention (CDC) reveal 66 percent of United States adults are overweight and of those, half are obese.

The overweight situation in the United States is so serious that the CDC has established a new initiative. Its primary national health objective is to reduce the percentage of obese adults from its current 34 percent of the adult population to 15 percent by the year 2010. The agency has created an extensive outreach program in an attempt to inform citizens of the health risks of obesity and being overweight. More than six thousand articles have appeared in the press explaining the perils, which mainly include:

1. Hypertension (high blood pressure)
2. Osteoarthritis (bone and cartilage degeneration)
3. Dyslipidemia (high cholesterol)
4. Type 2 Diabetes
5. Heart Disease
6. Stroke
7. Gallbladder Disease
8. Sleep Apnea and respiratory problems
9. Some Cancers (endometrial, breast, and colon)

Pretty frightening picture, right? Fortunately, the majority of you reading this book are probably not in serious danger, for you are not yet classified as obese, which is when the risk becomes imminent. Most individuals who have reached obesity levels are likely to be under a physician's care. However, the CDC does warn that merely being overweight can increase your exposure to these risks.

Social and Career Discrimination

The danger of being overweight, if not obese, extends beyond physical well-being. Excess weight often leads to personal and/or social distress and anxiety. In her book *Eating Disorders*, Dr. Hilde Bruch attributes this to "the obsession of the western world with slimness, the condemnation of any degree of over-weight as undesirable and ugly." Understanding the source of these emotions will allow for better control of feelings and weight issues, which is the focus of this book.

A 2006 study conducted for the Federal Ministry of Health in Germany concluded that feeling "fat" can be every bit as bad psychologically as actually being fat. While this study was done primarily with adolescents, my professional experience has shown it is 100 per-cent as applicable to adults as well. Even many of the respondents who were only moderately overweight stated that they forfeited a measure of quality of life because they believed they were "too fat."

Take Jane for example, a divorced client of mine who stands 5'3" and weighs 125 pounds. Recently, she made a comment that she had gained "almost 10 pounds" during the holidays. "I really feel fat now. So I'm not even going to try and date right now be-cause no guy would want me anyway!" she unhesitat-ingly exclaimed. Jane's remark is a prime example of how feeling fat overrides the reality of not being fat!

Researchers for the National Association to Advance Fat Acceptance (NAAFA) point out that victimization is a reality in the workplace as well. They found that 16 percent of the employers they polled stated that they would not hire an overweight woman. I suspect the percentage would possibly double if all employers were being totally honest. Researchers also claimed that salary levels of overweight men are reduced by an av-erage of $1,000 for each pound they are overweight.

The Weight-Loss "Industry"

Today, it is virtually impossible to read a newspaper, listen to the radio, or watch TV without being confronted by an advertisement or commercial touting a diet or exercise program guaranteeing that you <u>will</u> lose weight. This year, we can expect to see even more marketing efforts from the multi-million dollar weight-loss industry, inspired by government studies addressing the nation's obesity epidemic. In 2008, ad spending for weight-loss programs and products—excluding diet foods, diet beverages, and health clubs—totaled $241 million for the ten months between January and October, according to CMR/TNS Media Intelligence in New York.

Enticing photos, promises, and hard-sell texts are regularly used to convince you that weight loss can be achieved simply by following the prescribed plan. The "promised land" is within reach. Send in the prescribed fee, and rest assured, the pounds will disappear—as will your money! Just as important, programs guarantee that once you reach your goal, you will remain at that weight—just as the testimonial from the curvaceous female or sculpted male in the photograph says you will. Overall, commercial weight-loss programs virtually spend a scandalous number of dollars on claims that are not very believable even within the industry!

None other than Dr. Phil McGraw himself condemns these assurances as well. In his book, *The Ultimate Weight Loss Solution,* McGraw states, "Despite the millions of advertising dollars spent to convince you otherwise, losing weight and keeping it off is not 'quick and easy,' and you know it…you know it because you have been on umpteen diets…and not one of them has kept you slender."

Again, the "results not typical"/"results may vary" disclaimers reveal the true story. In fact, as you can probably tell, I become quite irritated every time I read those disclaimers—for they are really stating (in so many words) "let's face it folks: chances are this program won't work or it won't last!" The results obtained by most people who use the program surely, therefore, almost never equal those allegedly obtained by the testimonial-givers in the ads.

Studies Addressing Weight-Loss Programs

Recently, I assigned an assistant of mine to conduct an intensive search regarding any published studies of the success of weight-loss programs. She found three studies that seemed particularly relevant, all of which were published in the responsible and reputable *Journal of the American Medical Association.*

1. April 2003 – Results from Weight Watchers vs. a self-help program. The WW group did slightly better than those who did it on their own; but that, of course, was to be expected. Yet the amount of weight the WW group lost was on the average insignificant.

2. May 2005 – Atkins vs. Weight Watchers vs. Zone. The results were minimal weight losses in all three programs after dieting for one year.
3. March 2007 – Atkins vs. Ornish vs. Zone. Participants in all three programs lost only about ten pounds on the average by the end of one year.

Moral of the story? It appears from these studies that two not-very-inspiring conclusions are unavoidable. First, none of these well-touted programs appears to achieve any consistently better results overall than any other program. And second, none of these programs appears to achieve very good results by themselves... period. Not a very encouraging story, is it?

The "Missing Piece"

Often, people rush to slim down because of a forthcoming major life event, for example, a wedding, job interview, vacation, or the like. Looking for a quick solution, so many people immediately turn to the latest fad "diet du jour," or even to diet pills. Yet as you no doubt know from your own personal experience, these "quick fixes" aren't even guaranteed to work in the short run—and they virtually never work in the long run.

While the most current data supports my belief that diet and exercise alone is insufficient to reach your weight goal, the integral component omitted from almost all of these programs is, in my view, some type of *psychological counseling*. The rate of long-term weight-loss success can definitely increase when in addition to adhering to a diet and exercise plan, you also pursue some type of counseling for support. Consider this book one type of a "counselor" or "coach" on your personal journey to shed those excess pounds and keep them off once and for all!

Is There Truly Hope Here?

Yes there is, as you will discover in the chapters ahead. In addition to this book though, I'd like to mention there are few other books on the shelves of your local bookstore that also address psychological aspects of losing weight. Those especially worth the read are Dr. Judith Beck's *The Beck Diet Solution* and Dr. Roger Gould's *Shrink Yourself*.

My book on inner/psychological "blocks" to losing weight differs from these other books in that it offers a basic and straightforward method to addressing the inner negative forces that steer you to overeat and not exercise. My book especially teaches you how to tackle what will be characterized as the "Inner Bully," that is, everyone's symbolic internal "enemy" of self-control and self-discipline, and the source behind the self-sabotaging inner blocks presented in this book. You'll hear much more about your Inner Bully (IB) in the next chapter.

Hopefully, after reading this overview, there is at least some reassurance knowing you are in the company of millions, indeed billions around the globe, who struggle every day to lose weight. What certainly is <u>not</u> comforting on the other hand are the above-cited statistics highlighting the percentage of people who regain lost weight!

On that note, it's time for you to hear more about your "arch inner enemy," your Inner Bully.

Chapter 2
TACKLING YOUR INNER BULLY

* * *

When Jane arrived at my office one sunny morning, she initially appeared as cheerful and bright as the weather outside. The prototype of an overweight, borderline-obese woman in her mid thirties, Jane sat down, rifled through her purse, and handed me a photograph of herself. In the picture, Jane was slender, attractive, and seductively dressed. "This is what I looked like just three years ago," she said—and then proceeded to burst into uncontrollable tears. Once the initial torrent of tears passed, Jane shared her distressing history.

Shortly before the photograph was taken, Jane discovered her husband Dave had been cheating on her, with a good friend. She was deeply upset, because their marriage had seemed solid. When confronted, Dave begged forgiveness, insisting he loved Jane dearly, and promised to remain true. Although Jane accepted his assurance, she wanted a guarantee that he would be faithful. Throughout her life, whenever she sensed a problem in a relationship with a man, Jane blamed it on her weight. Once again, she felt her weight was the issue. Aware of having added some additional pounds during their early years of marriage, she assumed Dave was turned off by her size. Jane worked hard at slimming down, and ultimately succeeded, as proved by the photo. It, therefore, came as a devastating blow when she discovered his infidelity. Now believing her weight-loss efforts to be of no value, Jane returned to the fridge and pantry for solace and put back the pounds. Gaining substantial weight, she convinced herself divorce was inevitable, primarily because she was now "fat" again.

As though that were not enough for this despondent woman to bear, Jane lost her position as executive assistant to the CEO of an advertising agency when her boss retired. His replacement brought staff with him, and Jane was relegated to a lower-level job and a reduction in salary. Instead of acknowledging the real reason Jane lost the position, she again blamed it on her size. Surrendering to her uncontrolled food cravings, she continued to add more and more weight.

Almost ready to give up entirely, Jane met an old acquaintance while browsing the cookie counter in the local bakery. The friend proceeded to share and explain some of the work I was doing with inner blocks to weight loss. Feeling she had no other options, Jane set up an appointment and arrived at my office with reservation. She feared her inner fortitude to fight these self-sabotaging impulses simply did not exist.

Using the framework of the symbolic Inner Bully, I tailored a specific therapy program for Jane to address her specific self-sabotaging issues. Finally, she had a "real" enemy to challenge other than herself. As we worked together, Jane began to regard her IB as a negative force within her subconscious, separate from her conscious mind. This perspective enabled Jane to distance herself from her negative, weight-loss-sabotaging impulses. As a result, she no longer blamed herself for perceived weakness on the self-control front. Her IB became her "own worst enemy"—rather than herself. Months later, with sustained hard work and effort on both the eating-control and exercise fronts, Jane successfully reached her weight goal. She is now working at a new job, and has met a new male friend. Still in its early stage of bloom, Jane is not yet viewing this as a permanent or lifelong relationship. She, however, is enjoying the connection with this man, as well as—even more importantly—the restoration of her self-confidence!

Separating Yourself from Your Inner Bully

The advantage of my treatment program over most others is its central emphasis on tackling your IB—especially in order to help you break down your inner or psychological "Blocks" to losing weight. These so-called Inner Blocks (IBLs) are the major, selfsabotaging obstacles that your Inner Bully puts in place inside you in its never-ending quest to undermine your efforts on the weight-loss front. The potential IBLs that may be sabotaging you are the subject of Chapters 5 through 10 of this book. As a little sneak preview though, you will see that these blocks especially include self-rebellion, anxiety, loyalty issues, weight-loss "curse words," emotional deprivation/suppression, and spite.

As an aside, a thought or two regarding our sub-conscious mind is in order. Try thinking of it as functioning like an internal, invisible "computer." Then think of this computer as being split into two parts—at risk of oversimplifying matters, a positive part and a negative part. The positive part contains components that are of great psychological benefit to you, such as courage, willpower, determination, self-discipline, compassion, and empathy. When these elements are dominant, you are more able to function as a confident and contented human being, relate well to people, and generally maintain good self-discipline.

In contrast, the negative part of your "internal computer" harasses you with negative messages. How many times have you chastised yourself, ruminating about something you have eaten that has caused you to feel guilty? Perhaps it was finishing that whole quart of ice cream, or the unnecessary fueling of fat at a fast-food drive-in. Think of this negative part of your "computer" purely as a self-sabotaging mechanism, programmed to undermine your self-esteem and self-respect. Directed at you and you alone, it can blow out of proportion anything you perceive you have done out of weakness--in other words, involving loss of self-control. Your IB transmits these instant self-condemning messages directly from your subconscious. Functioning like a persistent "psychological virus," it causes you to feel you are never good enough to meet any challenge—especially losing weight. Since, however, you have now defined your "own worst enemy" as your IB rather than you, it is (as underscored above) essential to develop a separation from your IB, and recognize it as <u>the</u> source of all this negative input within you.

"Yeah, just keep on blowing your diet and look even uglier!" The more often your IB causes you to berate and criticize yourself with harsh words like these, the more vulnerable you become, not only to weight-loss sabotage, but also to *clinical* types of problems like depression and anxiety. These in turn can be accompanied by so-called psychosomatic symptoms, such as headaches, high blood pressure, gastrointestinal disturbances, and sleep impairment.

So even if you are just a little bit overweight, your IB can make you feel self-conscious, and lead you to perceive yourself as irredeemably fat. As it did for Jane, your IB's voice will send persuasive messages urging you to disregard your better judgment and seek consolation from sweets, carbs, or other scrumptious comfort foods. By serving as the conduit for these negative, self-undermining communications, your IB is just as menacing or vicious as any schoolyard bully—and harder to escape, since it "lives" invisibly inside you! Like the playground version, your IB follows, tracks, and attacks in every situation in which you are vulnerable.

What Motivates Your Inner Bully?

Since birth, your IB has been lurking inside your subconscious. Functioning as a life-long "sponge," in essence, it absorbs and stores away any and every judgmental or critical remark directed at you from your parents, siblings, other relatives, teachers, school-mates, and in later life, peers and bosses. No doubt, you've heard disparaging, demoralizing comments over the years like, "You'll never amount to anything!" or "You're stupid!" or "You're fat and ugly!" The list of these types of psychologically harmful comments is potentially endless.

Due to its long association within you, you can think of your IB as having adopted some of your personal characteristics—especially the content and tone of your speech. When the Bully talks to you inside your head therefore, it sounds as though the words and tone flow directly from you. Actually though, I advise you to think of your IB as a "master ventriloquist" within you. Pardon the pun, but your IB can leave you feeling like a real "dummy," for being fooled time and again into be-lieving that all of these mean-spirited, self-deprecating thoughts are really yours, rather than your Bully's!

The direct criticisms and belittlings leveled against you by your Inner Bully are not the only weapons in its arsenal. Another, more indirect set of weapons I call "sneak attacks" are used against you too by your ever-resourceful IB. Here are three examples.

First, we have *negative comparisons* with specific others, such as "Look at how much better Rhonda is doing in school than I am," or "Why can't I play tennis as well as Joe?" More relevantly to weight loss, you might think something like, "Why is Sandy so sleek and attractive, and I'm nothing but an unappealing chunk?" These negative comparisons likely echo similar types of statements that have been made to you over the years by others, most likely your parents or relatives. The comparisons, in turn, can reverberate in your mind, allowing the Bully to pummel you with them repeatedly.

A second "sneak attack" your IB can perpetrate against you is *perfectionism*. Perfectionists know that whatever you attempt to do, actually achieving perfection is…perfectly impossible! And then when the inability to achieve perfection leaves you disappointed or frustrated, your IB seizes the opportunity to drive you into discouragement, if not an outright, irrational sense of "failure." For example, John has lost most of the significant amount of weight he intended to lose (about fifty pounds)—but he still remains about ten pounds short of his goal. So what does he tell himself? Perfectionistically, John tells himself, "I just can't do it—I give up!" As a result, John proceeds to spend the next few weeks overeating to his heart's (mal)content.

Procrastination is a third type of "sneak attack" that your IB relishes using. The longer you put off starting a significant task like losing weight, the worse you will feel about yourself. You know you should tackle it, yet you manufacture a myriad of reasons to delay—all enthusiastically supported by the Bully. "Why did I wait to try and lose weight? Now I won't fit into the wedding dress" is a prime example of your IB scoring a victorious procrastinating "sneak attack" against you.

You can see from these examples what really happens in your "relationship" with your IB. Your negative feelings increase and depress you, but your IB feels proud it has accomplished its job. In fact, think of the primary purpose of your IB as trying to convince you that you <u>do not deserve</u> to get what you want in life—especially on the weight-loss front.

Managing the Two "Bs"—Your Bully and Your Binging

It is frustrating for me to hear my patients complain that friends or family members sometimes accuse them of being "masochists" because they have not been able to shed the pounds. I would not be surprised if you, too, have experienced a label like that at one time or another. Rest assured though, it is simply not true! A commonly misused term, Webster's Dictionary defines masochism as "the getting of pleasure, often sexual, from being hurt or humiliated." Masochism implies consciously and intentionally pursuing pain for pleasure—and so it is not applicable in this circumstance. The deceits and distortions that emanate from your IB <u>do</u> produce a degree of pain, unhappiness, and dissatisfaction. However, they are not inflicted by *you* against you.

Think about it. Have you ever planned to have self-deprecating condemnations enter your mind? Do you ever tell yourself, "Okay, in thirty seconds I'm going to place a very self-critical thought into my mind?" Of course not! Instead, self-degrading thoughts beyond your control suddenly "pop" into your mind from time to time. Planning self-belittlement would be masochistic; having these negative thoughts and self-perceptions spontaneously enter your thinking is not. So if you are not a masochist, why do you insist upon allowing the Bully to torment you?

Although you will never be able to rid yourself of your IB, you can learn to control it. You can teach yourself to cope and not respond to each of its self-deprecating messages.

The Four-Step Control Program

The recommended four-step program that follows will assist you in fighting back and better managing your IB in your quest to lose weight. This program applies both to maintaining eating-control at every meal and snack, as well as to getting exercise. Overall, it will help you strengthen your resolve to eat sensibly and exercise regularly, and resultantly reshape your overweight body into one of which you can be proud.

Step 1. Separation – Much of what I have stressed up to this point is the need to think of your IB as an entity totally separate from you. It becomes easier with practice to feel frustrated and irritated at "it"—and, therefore, oppose this inner negative "power"—than it is to skirmish with yourself. Once you are able to separate your IB and think of it as an enemy force within you, you will have a better chance to control it and significantly reduce its negative influence.

Step 2. Confrontation through Symbolism – When you have gained the confidence that separation makes possible, you will need to confront your IB's demands and temptations. This can be accomplished with practice by creating a concrete, tangible symbol for your

IB. To be utilized before any meal or snack, this symbol can help you with self-control over your eating, as well as used separately to help motivate you to exercise more regularly. The Bully's grasp on you can then gradually be diminished. But as you will see ahead, rebuffing your IB's instructions will take ongoing courage and determination on your part! (More on this use of symbolism in Chapter 4)

Step 3. Goal Setting – Setting goals for yourself are directly the opposite of what your IB has urged you to do. Three sets of goals worth setting are especially recommended: 1) goals regarding eating under control at every meal and every snack; 2) a goal regarding a realistic amount of exercise for you to do each week, based on number of days per week and number of minutes per day; and 3) a goal or two to work towards having nothing to do with weight loss, e.g., taking a class or two in some area of interest, doing some volunteer work, or finishing a project around the house (by doing so, you do not limit your need to succeed at something to only be losing weight, difficult a goal as that is of course to reach)

Step 4. Crediting Yourself – Give yourself the credit or acknowledgment you deserve for every positive step you complete. I especially recommend you develop the practice of reviewing the day's accomplishments each night. On days when you do well—that is, control your eating and do your exercise—take a few moments before going to sleep to reward yourself with a little verbal pat on the back, e.g., "You did really well today; way to go!" In other words, reinforce your determination to succeed by acknowledging and complimenting your efforts. Those beneficial thoughts will continue to reverberate in your mind long after you doze off, preparing you for another day of accomplishment. If you fall off the wagon though, simply label it a "detour," and then commit to getting back on track by the next day.

On that note, to the next chapter, which covers the important weight-loss-related subject of self-worth.

Chapter 3
WEIGHT LOSS AND SELF-WORTH

* * *

Each morning, I have a standing appointment for breakfast with Lou. Lou is not an exercise buddy or a business associate. Lou is my cat, who purringly eats his breakfast on the floor near my dining room table where I eat. I introduce you to Lou because Lou is a prime example of feeling comfortable with yourself—or at least appearing to anyway. Pets such as Lou can appear to have good self-esteem—even when, like my beloved Lou, they are in all honesty noticeably chunky!

Unlike Lou, most humans generally cannot be overweight and maintain good self-esteem at the same time. In addition, I think we can assume that overweight cats pay no price regarding their self-respect, whereas overweight humans do.

Self-Esteem, Self-Respect, and Self-Worth

The *New York Times* estimates that more than two thousand books have been written on the subject of self-esteem. Like individuals of all sizes and shapes, there are a myriad of definitions for the term *self-esteem*, as well as the term *self-respect.* Although people frequently use them interchangeably, these two terms are distinctly different in meaning. Yet, no matter how they are defined, these two personal qualities have a direct bearing on your efforts to lose weight, as well as on your ability to counter your IB's destructive pressures. They also, from my perspective, combine to form the following equation: self-esteem plus self-respect equals your overall emotional/psychological *self-worth*!

In his well-known description of the "Hierarchy of Needs," Abraham Maslow, father of Humanistic Psychology, included the individual's need for respect from others and the need for respect from one's self. Psychology professor and author Jennifer Crocker finds that, "People pursue self-esteem by trying to prove or demonstrate that they have worth and value." According to Nathaniel Branden, a noted author and expert on the subject, "Self-esteem is the experience of being competent to cope with the basic challenges of life and of being worthy of happiness." Unfortunately, too many definitions of self-esteem and self-respect involve comparison with others, and that's not healthy. As the well-known writer Joan Didion has said, "To free us from the expectations of others, to give us back to ourselves—there lies the great, singular power of self-respect." From my perspective, Didion can add overall self-worth as well.

<u>My</u> Definitions

Years of work with all types of patients has led me to create very specific definitions of self-esteem and self-respect that I use regularly. Starting with *self-esteem*, I define it as the positive personality character-istics and traits you possess which please you. In other words, self-esteem is what you like about yourself on the "inside."

I contrast that with my concept of *self-respect*, which I define as the sense of accomplishment you re-ceive from successfully pursued activities. These do not have to be major achievements however; your day-to-day "little" accomplishments are significant contribu-tors to your self-respect.

Just as the definitions of self-esteem and self-respect differ, these two states of mind generate dis-tinctively different emotional/psychological feelings internally. A high level of self-esteem is likely to be ac-companied by an optimistic sense of well-being. The higher the intensity, the greater the glow (i.e., "warm fuzzy") you will feel inside.

Self-respect in contrast engenders a less identifi-able, but more "foundational" response. People who possess a high level of self-respect know they've *earned* that feeling, through their persistent efforts and productive actions. The result is a good deal of self-confidence in most situations, and the development of a solid, core psychological base.

The combinations of these two mind-sets are key to helping you control your ongoing weight problem. It is essential that you understand how self-esteem and self-respect function and interact. If these qualities are not firmly established in you, the likelihood is that this could allow your IB to drive you to overeat and not exercise.

Physical Appearance and Self-Esteem

Visibly absent from this discussion regarding the definitions of self-esteem (and self-respect for that matter) are the words "physical appearance." This omission is intentional, and where I part company, especially, from what I think of as the "popular/traditional" definition of self-esteem.

For the majority of people, but especially for women, I firmly believe the degree of your self-perceived physical attractiveness plays a significant role in determining your level of self-esteem. An especially negative perception of your physical appearance becomes an important influence in diminishing your self-esteem—especially if you are overweight, much less obese. Therefore, in theory anyway, you must train your mind to dissociate your feelings about your physical appearance from your core, personality-based self-esteem. Of course, in practice this will be—need I tell you—a lot easier said than done!

As your core self-esteem increases, you will develop the strength to counter your IB's harmful negative impact on you, which involves trying to keep you disproportionally focused on how you feel about how you look on the *outside* compared to what you like about yourself on the *inside*. By working on reducing your assessment of your physical attractiveness as an element of your self-esteem, you can gradually cultivate the positive attitude essential to confront your IB, control momentary food cravings, and shed those extra pounds.

Accomplishing this separation most certainly will take time and effort! Regardless of your intelligence, personality, or motivation to complete this objective, if you are dissatisfied with your outward physical appearance, your negative feelings in this area will cloud your positive thoughts about your inner self. Therefore, from here on in, it is essential that you focus more on your positive/likable personality traits than you ever have before.

As a little aside, I am reminded at moments like this of a cartoon that terrifically captures the differential perceptions of physical attractiveness between the sexes. Without any caption, the cartoon contains two panels: one of an obese man, the second a shapely female. Each person is facing a full-length mirror. The paradox is that the slender woman sees reflected in the mirror a quite plump image of herself, while the heavy man sees a well-developed muscular "stud"! What could better portray the different relationship for men and women between self-perceived physical attractiveness and self-esteem than these cartoon images?

Building Up Your Self-Esteem and Self-Respect

Last but not least for this chapter, I highly recommend you cultivate more self-esteem and self-respect for yourself. On the self-esteem end, I especially encourage you to make a written list of any and all positive/likable personality traits and qualities you have that you are glad you have (e.g., loyalty, outgoingness, generosity, intelligence, and having a good sense of humor).

Then be sure to give yourself a nice little "boost" by reading over your list every day. That way, your force yourself to occasionally shift off focusing on—and negatively judging—your appearance on the outside, and shift on to what you really like about you on the inside. Or to put this slightly differently, start taking some of the "eggs" out of the primary "basket" of self-esteem that have mattered too much to you, and start putting them in a different, healthier "basket."

On the self-respect front, how about making sure at the end of the day you take a minute or so to remind yourself of anything you accomplished that day, big or little. In other words, whether it's something big (like completing a major job assignment), or something "little"(like exercising that day), make sure you give yourself a bit of self-credit where credit is due. After all, if *you* don't give some credit to yourself where it's due, who else can you assume will?

Now to an overview of what I view as your IB's primary undermining "attack measures" it uses against you—your IBLs (Inner Blocks) to losing weight.

Chapter 4
THOSE SELF-SABOTAGING "INNER BLOCKS"

* * *

Introduction

It's January 1 and time to establish your New Year's resolutions. What could be more pressing than the desire to lose weight? You vow to lose fifteen pounds by Cousin Sue's wedding in March, followed by another ten for the opening of the summer swim season in mid-June. You are so determined to succeed that you boldly declare your intention to your circle of people closest to you.

You set tomorrow as launch day for your new diet and personally designed daily exercise plan. Don't expect to catch your IB "off duty" though. Always on the alert, your IB quickly bombards you with a menu of excuses to postpone the start of your program (a la the procrastination "sneak attack"). If you do somehow muster up the strength to resist its dictates and begin, your IB will be ready and willing all along the way to disrupt your progress.

Your willpower may temporarily be so strong that you remain disciplined in spite of your IB's sabotaging attacks on you. As you come within a few pounds of your first weight-loss goal, you haven't let the Bully derail your purpose—until now that is. For example, suppose you have a disagreement with your supervisor at work. Upset, you miss a day of exercise and mitigate your feelings with a "small" serving of cake, topped with vanilla ice cream. From there, you slip into a second bad day, followed by a third, until it's just a matter of time before you give up. Gradually you regain most if not all of the weight lost.

You are not alone sharing this weight-loss pattern. Weighing in at 245 pounds, five-foot-eight Jim felt ill after binging throughout the holiday season. He finally decided to trim down to the tight, muscular body he enjoyed as a college football star. In two months, Jim lost twenty pounds. However, Jim became distraught when the company he worked for was sold and the new group announced relocation of its headquarters to North Dakota. As a result, Jim ended up overindulging the contents of his snack drawer. His resolve flew away, perhaps to North Dakota, but his remaining 225 pounds stayed in Pennsylvania, and soon returned to their original level.

Erica's experience was different. A bridesmaid for her best friend Jill, Erica had been told a good-looking young man was coming to San Francisco from the East Coast to attend the wedding. A bit overweight, Erica wanted to eliminate the extra few pounds. She felt confident that she could accomplish her goal in the seven weeks prior to the wedding, at which time she was to be paired with the "cute" groomsman. The diet was proceeding on track until Erica had lunch with a co-worker one afternoon. Sharing her resolution, Erica munched on her salad and described her three weeks of progress using a vegetarian diet. Casually remarking there wasn't a noticeable difference in Erica's shape, the co-worker concluded that Erica would not reach the goal. Erica's IB emerged to lower her resistance, and marked the end of the diet and exercise routines.

This up-and-down cycle, as you well know, can become a chronic pattern. The result is a sort of contradiction in terms, but only on the surface. You "gain" something—weight; but you also "lose" something— self-esteem and self-respect—though your goal is to achieve the exact opposite. Or to state this in IB language, your IB wins, while you fail!

Uncovering Your Inner Blocks

A publication by The Cleveland Clinic Bariatric and Metabolic Institute states that only about 1 percent of all cases of obesity are believed to be caused by certain medical conditions. Therefore, unless you have a health-related condition or you are on a medication triggering weight gain as a side effect, you can assume that you have one or more self-sabotaging, psychological obstacles that block you from losing weight and keeping it off. These IBL's are put in place by your (who else) IB, for the sole purpose of sabotaging your resolution to lose weight. To be able therefore to lose weight and then keep it off, these IBLs need to be identified and controlled. Recognizing the root cause of each Block will help you begin to break down that particular Block, and may, in time, significantly reduce your vulnerability to all of the negative pressures exerted by your IB.

As individuals, each person will experience different IBLs. In other words, we've got a case here of "different strokes for different folks"—and so I will be devoting the remaining chapters of this book to a description of <u>all</u> of the possible Blocks. Over the many years of my practice, I have found that in most instances there are several IBLs at work within the same person. It is even possible for a single individual to possess all six of the Blocks covered ahead! You will have to decide which one or more of them applies specifically to you.

Tackling Your Inner Blocks through IB Symbolism

So how can you achieve control of your IBLs to lose weight? While it is not an easy task, it is not impossible either. Most importantly, you will have to make a concerted and mindful effort to challenge your self-sabotaging IB , before every meal and every snack. You will recall that back in Chapter 2, I mentioned a key method of controlling your IB is through symbolism. Let's take a more thorough look at this technique.

The first step is choosing an effective *symbolic object* for your IB. Whether you select a drawing, a photograph, or a small physical object to use as a symbol, it must have an unpleasant-looking, "bully-ish" appearance. Some of my patients have chosen an evil spirit, such as a demon or a devil. Others have used photos of an angry person or a ferocious animal, while others have chosen a small troll-like creature that fits in the palm of your hand. Make your choice carefully, and be sure that it connects you immediately in your mind to your troublemaking IB.

Next, your symbolic object needs a tormenting caption or two, which reinforces your determination to confront your Bully. Fire up your creative skills, and craft a message that captures what your IB might say to you if it was a an actual real-life bully—in this case trying to bully you into eating more than you should or things you shouldn't. Here are a few examples of such captions I'd recommend you consider using:

"Go ahead, you loser—you have no control anyway!"

"What a liar you are about wanting to lose weight!"

"I'm in control here, not you!"

"Come on, who cares about self-esteem and self-respect!"

Once chosen or designed, your symbolic object and its tormenting captions remain with you at all times. Keep them in your purse or wallet—after all, the likelihood of finding food and a reason to eat is always present. Here's the key though: just before any meal or snack, take out your object and captions, and concentrate on them for about fifteen to thirty seconds. Then let your justifiable resentment and frustration take over. In your mind, confront your IB symbol with some blunt words like, "Back off right now and don't tell me what to do or think!" or "I'm staying in control; the heck with you!" You must then immediately proceed to eat only what you should and no more than you should—or else your efforts to focus on your symbolic object and accompanying captions will be undermined. Use a similar two-part symbolic technique on days you find yourself shying away from doing your exercise.

By weakening the grip of your IB in this symbolic yet blunt manner, you can (with lots of practice of course) effectively control your food choices better and get more regular exercise. By doing so, you can then, in turn, focus your attention mainly on those IBLs that "roadblock" your weight-loss efforts.

On now to the next chapter, where I begin an analysis of the six specific possible Blocks, starting with the most universal and troublesome one of all—what I call "addiction to self-rebellion."

Chapter 5
INNER BLOCK NUMBER ONE: ADDICTION
TO SELF-REBELLION

* * *

Have you ever thought of yourself as a "rebel?" Maybe not in quite a while, if ever. Yet if you are unable to control your intake of food and you don't exercise regularly, then I suggest you start considering yourself a specific type of rebel: a weight-loss rebel! Like so many others who cannot seem to take off weight and keep it off, it is time to ask, "What or whom am I rebelling against?" The answer is mainly against yourself, and your own best interests concerning weight loss. Secondarily though, you may be rebelling against any family members and friends who, although they care about you, nonetheless often pressure you to lose weight. As a result, you can become frustrated with them because they don't seem to understand that years of experience have shown you just how a tough a battle losing weight really is! So you end up overeating and not exercising almost out of a subconscious spite against this pressure. I will discuss more on spite as a secondary type of rebellion against losing weight in Chapter 10.

Sally's case is a classic illustration of this very type of two-pronged rebellion. Sally had great trouble controlling her overindulgent eating. Waking up each morning, her first trip was directly to the refrigerator—rather than say to a local health club. Only 5'2", Sally weighed 176 pounds, far too heavy for her frame. In addition, Sally had to contend with her mother's frequent haranguing about her weight. This only made Sally angrier and more determined than ever to continue overeating—in the process rebelling against both herself as well as her mother, as though "killing two birds with one (rebellion) stone," you might say.

Webster's dictionary defines a rebel as one who "resists any authority or established usage." As you consider this definition, your thoughts undoubtedly turn to the actions of an adolescent or young adult, perhaps someone you knew growing up in your neighborhood or your school. If you are old enough, James Dean, the personification of the classic "rebel without a cause," may come to mind. Then again, maybe the prime example for you of a rebel is: the kid you saw in the mirror each morning?

If you were like many kids growing up, you may have rebelled at times against rules you did not like, and against the people who made the rules. Of course, if those rule-makers were your parents, you loved them but still resented their rules, given the "rigidity" and "meanness" you felt your parents exhibited when they demanded that you actually follow their rules.

As a little aside, if you think about it though, rebellion isn't always a negative behavior. It can also involve standing up and asserting yourself for a cause in which you strongly believe (e.g., as portrayed by Sally Field in the role of Norma Rae, in the movie by that name about oppressive workplace conditions). That is something we can all respect. Although some people may not particularly like your style or persistence, there still is room to acknowledge and appreciate your courage and determination when you demonstrate conviction about your rebellious-appearing cause.

In the case of weight loss, in contrast, the fact that you feel you have struggled to limit your food intake and get some exercise, but are unable to do so, no doubt triggers a great deal of frustration and disappointment in you. These negative emotions, in turn, lead you to rebel, but in a purely self-defeating way—encouraged of course by your ever-present IB, who as you know by now thrives on steering you to sabotage your physical and mental well-being.

A Preferred Definition of Rebellion

My preferred definition of rebellion as it relates to weight loss differs from Mr. Webster's. Comprised of two parts, rebellion can first be defined as anything you do that involves doing the opposite of what's in your *best interest*. Secondly though, rebellion is anything you do that involves doing the opposite of what you feel *overly pressured* to do by significant others. On the latter front, you may be aware that it is to your advantage to follow their advice and admonitions regarding your self-control and self-discipline, looking at things logically. Unfortunately, what you refuse to face is that in the end, it is you and your welfare that you're really rebelling against, more than anything and anyone in particular.

Each and every time you eat more than you should, or eat something you shouldn't, or find an excuse not to exercise, face it...you are rebelling! Then, complicating matters further, you are knowingly sabotaging yourself by finding rationalizations for this behavior. For example, following a difficult day at work, you may feel the need for a stress-reliever or simply a little pleasure. So you reach into your trusty panty, refrigerator, or candy drawer and proceed to overindulge yourself with tasty morsels of food—in spite of how well you've been doing of late on your chosen diet. This rebellious pattern may also hold true in the aftermath of feeling "scolded" for your overindulgences, by, say, your spouse, romantic partner, friend, boss, or even your physician.

Why would you ever want to do exactly the opposite of what you know is in your best interest? If you answer, "Because I must be a masochist," let me point out, as explained in a previous chapter, that no one consciously and consistently attempts to do the opposite of what is in his/her best interest—no one! In fact, in any aspect of life—not just on the weight-loss front—when we do the opposite of what is in our best interest, we do it automatically and reflexively, with little if any conscious thought involved. In other words, we do it on *impulse*—then basically watch our good judgment go right out the window in the process!

How many times have you intended to eat a salad instead of a burger and fries, but you still went ahead and ordered the burger/fries combo? How often have you set a limit of say a half a cup of ice cream after dinner, and then devoured about half a gallon? On the exercise front, I'm sure you can remember times you were determined to exercise sometime that day, but then manufactured an excuse not to follow through. In each of these instances, you acted on impulse in a self-defeating way, against your best interest. You willingly made the wrong choice, assuming of course that you wanted to lose weight and keep it off. So why keep making the wrong choice?

You are not deliberately trying to sabotage your weight-loss efforts. Something within you, in your subconscious, compels you to do this, thwarting all of your good intentions. That "something" you can assume is the combination of your sabotaging IBLs plus your spiteful IB, teaming up against you over and over!

Rebellion And The Trouble-Making "Shoulds"

Consider instances when you were tempted to rebel and surrendered. Each time, you ignored the warning that your IB had begun its efforts at sabotage. You can greatly improve your chance of outwitting your IB by responding to that early signal. The hint is in your internal, spontaneous use of the word "should," or slight variations, like "ought to," "have to," or "supposed to." Those words entering your mind provide notice that your IB is about to sabotage you on the eating and/or exercise fronts. For example, envision yourself deciding whether to eat a fruit platter or a bowl of nachos for lunch. Logically, you will tell yourself that you "should" select the healthy platter, but you choose the nachos instead. Or hear yourself saying in your mind you really "should" exercise that day, but then you don't. Unlike when you tell yourself you "must" eat the fruit platter and you "must" exercise, your emphasis on the word "should" indicates that you actually are wavering, which in turn provides an opening for the Bully to lead you down the wrong path.

Think about the word "should" a bit more. It has other negative connotations as well, especially when used in an authoritarian-sounding manner. Telling yourself that you really "should" do something— whatever that something might be, and no matter how beneficial to you it might be—can sound a lot like a "lecturing parent" is speaking to you. You feel pressured to comply with this parental-sounding order. As a result though, this triggers in you an immediate and automatic switching into what I can only call a "rebellious kid." Or to put this slightly differently, self-rebellion, sparked by self-sabotaging "should-type" thoughts that enter your mind, is then played upon by your IB. So you end up telling yourself in so many words, "What the heck, I'll just get back on my diet tomorrow. I've been good for the last few days, so I can treat myself this one time!" At which point the "rebellious kid" takes over in you, and you go right ahead and eat more than you should and/or something you shouldn't! The same basic rebellious process also occurs of course when you try and "should" yourself into exercising Etcetera, etcetera, etcetera.

As a little aside, if you have any question regarding the validity and accuracy of what I have described about self-rebellion, I recommend you go ahead ask someone trying to lose weight how they fared that day. If he/she admits, "Well, I must confess, I really slipped pretty badly today!" watch for a smile, embarrassed giggle, or nervous laugh that almost inevitably follows. The large majority of people who admit on that particular day they either ate more than they should, ate something they shouldn't, or didn't exercise almost always, I find, react with a guilty smile, often enough accompanied by a chuckle. This, if you think about it, is basically the same reaction you are likely to get from a young rebellious kid when caught in a convenient lie!

So whether the ambiguity of "should" gives the Bully more ability to control you or the word's authoritarian nature reminds you of a lecturing parent, you will take the path of self-rebellion. Acting in opposition of your best interests, you sabotage yourself, in the process insisting (in so many words), "Hey, don't tell me what to do. Because I'll just go ahead and do what I really want to do!" Once again, your IB is victorious, and you are defeated. Chances are though that you're not actually going to feel like a "loser" at that moment, as you indulge in a sumptuous slice of chocolate cake or a heaping portion of pasta smothered in cream sauce. In a similar vein, since exercise isn't much fun for most people, there is not likely to be a sense of disappointment when you bypass training that day. Yet you will in fact be a certain type of loser all right—just not of weight! Whether you admit it to yourself or not, your self-respect diminishes each and every time you go astray. If you then remain off-target or fluctuate between being in and out of self-control, you end up losing even more self-respect—not to mention self-esteem as well. This cycle continues in a downward spiral, for you and your overall self-discipline.

Eventually, you also lose something else—credibility. After all, why should anyone believe your expression of commitment to controlling your eating and getting regular exercise when they often instead see you doing the exact opposite? Eventually, you no longer believe it yourself. After all, your "actions speak louder than words," don't they? You, therefore, owe it to yourself to realize that your weight-loss rebellious actions often contradict your weight-loss words!

Your "Addiction" to Rebellion and How to Curb It

The type of rebellion discussed above pretty much assumes many of the characteristics of an *addiction*, because it occurs with such regularity. You may immediately think of the more common forms of addiction, like alcoholism and drug abuse, and protest that no one can accuse you of being an "addict." *Webster's Dictionary* basically defines addiction as being devoted yet surrendered to something habitual or obsessive. My definition of addiction however is broader, i.e., addiction is any behavior that is in control of you rather than vice versa, which results in psychological, physical, or financial harm to you, and/or to one of your relationships. Certainly, ongoing rebellion that manifests itself in your pattern of overeating and under-exercising fits this meaning of addiction all too well. Throw in the fact that you do not absolutely have to drink alcohol or use drugs to live, but you do have to eat to live, and you frankly end up with an even bigger challenge trying to control a food addiction than with any other type of substance addiction!

Overall, a shift in your priorities must first take place. Your goal of losing weight now needs to focus on breaking down your IBL's. Managing your food intake better will follow automatically once you've gradually gained control over these inner "saboteurs." Similarly, you will discover that regular exercise becomes a part of your weekly routine.

Best of all, if you are following one of the advertised diet or exercise plans that are often ineffectual, it will become easier to comply with the plan, and thus may produce more dramatic results in the long run!

All of this becomes easier if you gradually teach yourself to heed the early "should" warnings and immediately utilize the symbolic object you have previously chosen to counter the undermining force of the Bully. (Remember, we discussed symbolism as a mechanism to control your IB at the end of the last chapter.) By following this routine, you will, in effect, pre-empted your IB before its rebellion-creating, self-sabotaging messages can sway you to violate the weight-loss commitments you have made. Or to put this a bit differently, it's time to work on controlling your "lecturing parent" from "should'ing" you into evoking (and provoking) your "rebellious kid" into action—and instead just concentrate on maintaining the self-control and self-discipline of a…responsible adult!

Last but not least, I cannot guarantee that this strategic and consistent focus on controlling your self-rebellion Block alone will cure your eating problems and get you to exercise more regularly. A number of other IBLs can sabotage your efforts in addition to addiction to self-rebellion. They are the subject of the remaining chapters in this book. Just remember that you can experience more than one IBL at any given time. Self-rebellion is the universal Block, and that is why I have begun with it. But it may join forces with one or more other IBLs. If you find yourself falling off your plan, be honest enough to face that other factors inside of you besides self-rebellion also might be keeping you from losing weight and keeping it off. The following chapters will help you do that.

Postscript "Food For Thought": Exercises

1. List the circumstance under which you are most likely to rebel on the weight-loss front. For example, are some foods more difficult to control than others? Are you most likely to eat more than you should at meals, snacks, or special occasions—or all of the above?

2. What reactions from others trigger your rebellion?

3. On a scale of one to five, how much of a rebel are you when it comes to exercising?
4. Aside from eating and exercising, are there any other areas of your life in which you tend to be a rebel?
5. For the next week, make a brief entry in a notebook describing what you felt five minutes after you ate something you shouldn't have, or ate more than you should have.

Chapter 6
INNER BLOCK NUMBER TWO: ANXIETY

* * *

Let's take a look now at *anxiety*, the second of the six IBLs to weight loss. This Block exerts a wide reach, and can sabotagingly weave its way into many different aspects of your life, as you will see from the case studies in this chapter. Hearing this, you may scratch your head and wonder, "Can anxiety really affect the success or failure of my effort to lose weight?" The answer is that it surely can, and you're about to see the ways it can play such a powerful role, as we probe deeper into what is happening inside your subconscious.

You are about to discover that anxiety can create a pattern within you of "approach/avoidance" (to be discussed below), spurred on by the urgings of your IB. The following three case studies illustrate, in different ways, the pervasiveness of this anxiety Block to losing weight. They will also help you look at your own anxieties, and how they are, in all likelihood, negatively affecting your efforts to lose weight and keep it off.

Dara's Dilemma

Dara was a woman in her early forties who had grown increasingly unhappy in her marriage of eight years. She continued to feel dependent on her husband Jerry, both financially and emotionally, part of which was the result of the extra forty pounds she carried on her frame. Although she was intelligent and personally likable, Dara was quite insecure and uneasy about the prospect of a marital separation and ultimate divorce, and thus ending up living her life alone.

Complicating matters for Dara was the fact that Jerry loved her very much. His devotion to her was often smothering, but was something she appreciated, at least for its sincerity. In addition, she recognized that, like herself, Jerry was quite insecure; therefore, wanted to spare him from the hurt of a separation. Yet the fact was, for quite some time, Dara had found herself falling out of love with Jerry. She had particularly been unable to tolerate his lack of ambition, social aloofness, irresponsibility with money, and deep over attachment to his mother—none of which she was convinced had a chance of ever changing.

To make matters worse, Dara recently found herself strongly attracted to a handsome and personable co-worker named Ron. She began to fantasize about being with Ron—in every sense of the term "being"—something she had never done in her eight years of marriage. Each time Dara slipped into exciting daydreams about Ron, she came to an abrupt halt when she reminded herself of those forty or so extra pounds on her body. It was impossible for Dara to imagine that Ron, or any other man for that matter, could truly desire her because of her size.

Dara came to realize that going ahead and shedding those extra pounds had become a two-edged sword. On the one hand, she recognized she would become more attractive to a man like Ron; and as a result, her self-esteem and self-confidence would certainly build. On the other hand, Dara knew if she thinned down that she would feel more tempted to "cross the line"—but she also knew that Jerry would be devastated if he discovered that she was having an affair.

Dara thus found herself in a real quandary. Losing weight would certainly please her and make her feel enough of a gain in her self-esteem to feel more attractive to other men like Ron. But it inevitably would expose her to temptation, and potentially jeopardize her marriage—the prospect of which, at this point in her life, made Dara very anxious, no matter how dissatisfied she was staying married to Jerry. Dara's response to this core dilemma was to continue sabotaging her efforts to lose weight. Instigated by her IB, an uncontrollable impulse to overeat overtook Dara. Stated another way, Dara became very anxious inside about being unable to control her impulses to have an affair, about the prospect of hurting Jerry, and about the prospect of living out on her own if the marriage ultimately ended. As a result of these different but related anxieties, Dara ended up making certain she would remain undesirable to other men, by remaining overweight!

Dave's Difficulty

Dave's dream when he graduated from high school was to become a lawyer. He majored in Political Science in college, and applied to several law schools. His overall grade-point average in college was not exceptional, and the fact that he struggled with standardized entrance exams led to rejections from those few law schools to which he applied. Dave internalized this rejection. He lost much of the self-confidence he had always possessed—even while going through college carrying an additional fifty-five pounds on his frame. Dave began to blame his self-defined failures on his weight. Instead of buckling down and reapplying to law school the following year, Dave took a self-imposed personal sabbatical for approximately six months. During that period, he spent much of the time in relative seclusion, basically ashamed of his appearance. Subsequently, Dave applied for and eventually accepted a "safe" entry-level position with the government.

Dave never abandoned the desire to become a lawyer. Meanwhile, over the years, he gradually rose in civil service ranking in his government position. He liked the security and the benefit package provided by the job. The nine-to-five work schedule was a welcome bonus as well. Yet Dave continued to dream of becoming an attorney someday, even if he found it too difficult to give up his desk job—especially because it protected him from having to interact with strangers outside of the office, a possibility that made Dave very anxious indeed.

One day, Dave's best friend Lance shocked him. Lance announced his plan to leave a well-paying engineering job over the next year while training to become a chef, a passion and career he had always wanted to pursue. Lance then proceeded to challenged Dave, saying "Hey Dave, if I have the guts to make this big career change, why don't you try to attend law school at night?"

Unfortunately, Dave could not find the courage to make such a bold move. As he wrestled with his thoughts, Dave reminded himself that a large part of his complacency in his safe government position was not having to leave his office and deal with the public. It was a way to avoid feeling self-conscious about his weight. In addition, Dave's confidence in his intelligence had never quite recovered from earlier rejections by the law schools to which he had applied.

Overall, Dave faced a similar type of tug-of-war inside that had stymied Dara. On the one hand, he knew if he took off the fifty extra pounds, he would gradually feel better about himself, restore some of his self-esteem, and maybe even eventually be comfortable with the public appearances he would have to face if he ever became a lawyer. On the other hand, Dave knew if he lost weight he would no longer have an excuse to avoid studying for and taking the law school entrance exams, a disconcerting thought for someone with so little confidence in his basic intelligence.

Inevitably, Dave regained whatever weight he had lost. As a result, he never again applied to law school and, therefore, stayed in his safe government job.

Unlike his friend Lance, Dave lived with regret every day because he had allowed his IB to use his anxiety Block as a way to avoid making the career move that could have changed his life.

Susie's Saga

Congenial and accomplished, Susie moved through life harboring a secret she never shared with anyone, including her significant other Marty. Now in her early forties, Susie had never sought professional help for the unhealed emotional "wound" inside her caused by several years of sexual molesting by her stepfather, which began when she was eight years old. Until she met Marty, Susie had bounced from one unhealthy romantic relationship to another, and remained significantly overweight throughout most of her adult years.

This childhood trauma of molestation left an indelible mark on Susie. Yet she managed to shield it from others, including the men with whom she had the closest relationships. An active and capable sex partner, Susie acted as though she enjoyed sexual relations, when in fact she never once reached orgasm—except when alone and self-stimulating.

After a number of unrewarding affairs, Susie met Marty, who also was overweight. A very loving person, Marty never hesitated to demonstrate his fondness for Susie. He had no problem with Susie's size and found her an ideal romantic partner. Susie felt very fortunate to have found him. Their sex life was fine, at least on the surface. Marty regularly enjoyed orgasm, and Susie frequently faked it so that Marty would not feel inadequate. Nevertheless, even though they became very close, Susie felt she could not share her secret with Marty. She convinced herself he would find her "dirty"—irrational as this was—and thus end the relationship.

Since Marty never complained about her size or gave her the impression he wanted her to lose weight, Susie remained complacent in her overweight "nirvana." She also continued to tell herself that her inability to reach orgasm was solely the result of her size, not her childhood trauma. Overall, Susie's core anxiety about experiencing true sexual intimacy with a partner provided the impetus that her IB used to steer her to keep binging and remain overweight.

Your Turn

Now that you have seen some ways anxiety can block people from achieving their goal of losing weight, it's time to look at your own situation. This requires your candid and objective effort. Specifically, you need to be totally honest with yourself as you answer the following question: "Is there anything that I am anxious about regarding my losing weight?"

To explore this a little deeper, let's look at how each of the case studies presented relates to the question I had you ask yourself. Are you, for example, experiencing the kind of relationship-related anxiety that plagued Dara? Perhaps you're more in tune with Dave's job and school-related anxieties? Or is there perhaps any correlation between what disturbs you and Susie's sexual and intimacy-related anxieties? Or is it possible that you are experiencing an entirely different category of anxiety that you lack the courage to tackle, unrelated to Dara's, Dave's, or Susie's?

Regardless of the specific anxiety you may be avoiding facing, it is magnified and used against you by your IB. There is no escape. Your anxiety serves as the ammunition your IB needs to sabotage your weight-loss efforts. As a result, you shy away from acknowledging and addressing your anxiety, refuse to help yourself or obtain professional counseling, and continue to use the refrigerator or cupboard as your "best friend." Your Bully has convinced you that remaining overweight allows you to avoid facing your underlying fears and to sidestep the task of bringing them under control.

"Approach-Avoidance" Conflict

"Approach-avoidance" conflict, as it is called, has been studied for years by psychological researchers. Let me refer you to studies conducted by two eminent psychologists back in the mid-twentieth century in particular. Drs. John Dollard and Neal Miller conducted experiments with laboratory rats, in the days before animal rights organizations and other watchdog groups closely monitored animal experiments. The two researchers placed hungry white rats at the start of a runway constructed appropriate to their size. The rats sprinted down the runway searching for their "treasure," a dish of food. Dollard and Miller continued this pattern repeatedly until the rats clearly learned that their hunger would be allayed at the far end of the runway.

However, this "no-brainer" of an invitation to a meal ended when Dollard and Miller began to administer electric shocks to the rats at a point when they neared the food dish. Suddenly "mealtime" changed radically for the ravenous rats. Specifically, the pattern became: the rats would continue to sprint toward their goal, but they would stop abruptly whenever they reached the point of having been shocked. Backing up a little, they would try again to move forward, sometimes racing, and other times approaching gingerly. But in each case, as they approached the "shock spot," the rats again shifted into reverse, and back-pedaled. This back-and-forth routine persisted until they neared starvation. The rats were then removed from the runway and fed. This experimental description shows how and why this situation is labeled "approach-avoidance" conflict.

The Human A-A Syndrome

Do you see the correlation between the Dollard/ Miller experiments on rats and the difficulty so many people face in losing weight? As most humans head down the "runway" to losing weight, a "shock to the system" can occur. For Dollard and Miller's rats, the shock was a literal one. In humans trying to lose weight, the "shock" can be the anxiety Block rearing its head. That especially applies when well-intentioned people like you begin the "roller-coaster ride" of losing and regain-ing weight—up and down the scale for us, back and forth in the runway for the rats.

When we move from the reactions of four-legged rats to analyzing approach-avoidance conflicts in our own two-legged population, something else is evident that differentiates us. That is, people can develop anxi-ety problems by simply *thinking* about an issue. It is not necessary for human beings to experience directly the kind of shock the rats underwent in order to begin fretting and worrying over something that can distress us—such as losing weight. Conversely, at times we are able to avoid a distressing situation because it can be anticipated. That anticipation may in turn lead to a constructive effort. You feel motivated to approach and solve the problem before it blossoms into a Block—and, therefore, before your IB can launch another sabotag-ing campaign. If and when you can achieve that de-gree of awareness and self-control, you will be well on your way to approaching—and only approaching—a successful weight-loss program!

Resolving Anxiety Blocks

Just as there are many causes of anxiety Blocks, different antidotes exist to neutralize them. Be aware though that most of all, anxiety-Block management re-quires courage. This quality will lead you to address anything that you are reluctant or hesitant to address, but you know that it is in your best interest to do so anyway—especially related to losing weight.

Let's take a few minutes now to see how the three cases outlined earlier might have ended in positive ways with courage in place.

Dara

Consider the courage Dara had to muster up when she actually began an intensive program to trim her weight, despite her concern over possibly separating from and hurting Jerry. For example, she could have agreed to see a marriage counselor, to address the issues that troubled her about her relationship with Jerry. As a result of the counseling, Dara might have developed enough inner fortitude to recognize that Jerry's assumed dependence on her may actually have been an exaggeration in her own mind, stemming from her own earlier marital needs.

Dara's courage and resilience would have helped her manage any guilt she had about hurting her former loved one. She would recognize that Jerry had many options for comfort, help, and support—from family, friends, therapists, and support groups. Focused more now on the potential fulfillment her new life, Dara could then look in the mirror and see clearly, and excitedly, that the physical image of herself she had hoped for had been achieved. No longer would she have to fear that she was unappealing inside or out. With a new figure, renewed self-esteem, and heightened self-respect, Dara would feel confident enough to move on with her life without Jerry. In the process, she would outmaneuver her IB; the sense of accomplishment she reaped, in theory, should keep her Bully (and former anxiety Block) under control for a very long time.

Dave

Risk-taking was Dave's psychological "weak spot." Even when goaded by his closest friend, Lance, to make a major life transition, Dave's resolve faded. As noted previously, using his weight as an excuse, Dave allowed his IB's arguments to be internalized and, therefore, believed he was unattractive, unappealing, and unworthy.

Specific goals could have been established and attained if Dave had possessed the courage and desire to change his life. He might, for example, have gone back to school to prepare for another round of examinations, or perhaps even chosen to become a paralegal. Even if he chose to abandon his dream of entering the legal profession, Dave could have created a solid résumé to search for a new, more challenging job. A visit to a job placement professional just might have helped Dave realize his potential.

The key to overcoming Dave's type of anxiety Block is tackling anxiety-producing specific goals one at a time. Each accomplishment will lead to greater confidence and strength to confront your IB. As the cycle begins to work, increased confidence leads to better self-esteem and then improved self-respect. In Dave's case, his spirit could have improved, and he would have been able to share his new career plans with close friends and family. Their support, in turn, would have reinforced his courage and determination. In addition, a simple but effective tool for someone like Dave is to *reward* himself, with a real pat on the back at the end of every productive day, along the lines of "way to go man, you really did well today!" This would have helped build Dave's confidence, as his subconscious mind mulled over his successes—on the career front and on the weight-loss front—while he slept.

Susie

Susie's situation can be viewed as more challenging than the other two. Overcoming anxiety about unresolved sexual issues and traumatic childhood experiences can be an extremely painful process. The weight problem that she used as an "avoidance cushion," so to speak, was only a minor part of the problems she had to face. Bottom line: Susie needed to muster up the courage to visit a professional counselor. Under his/her guidance, Susie would likely become better equipped to face those issues and experiences and the anxieties they produce, without severe harm to her psyche. With professional help Susie would be able to gradually overcome the anxiety Block that undermined her sexual gratification with the partner of her dreams, which in turn likely would free her up to eventually lose weight.

In Closing

In closing, I suggest you pull all of the information presented in this chapter together and get to work on conquering your underlying anxieties interfering with your ability to lose weight and keep it off. No matter what your specific anxieties are, you must shift out of the approach-avoidance "roller-coaster" cycle that your IB has reinforced, and into a real commitment to courage and honesty with yourself. It will take resolving these anxieties to begin a lifestyle that keeps you on the committed path to eating healthy and toning your body, while in the process building up your confidence, self-esteem, and self-respect.

I am certain you will concur that the rewards will be totally worth your courageous efforts!

On that note, on to the next weight-loss Block—what I call body image "curse words."

Chapter 7
INNER BLOCK NUMBER THREE:
BODY IMAGE "CURSE WORDS"

* * *

Terminology plays a major role in any weight-loss program. The words you use to describe your body image can set the tone and determine the success or failure of your efforts. These words can be discouraging and depressing, or they can be encouraging and uplifting. Let's look at some examples of both, but especially the former, which I characterize as weight loss "curse words."

The "F-Word"

Just as it is in street jargon, the use of an "f-word" is common in weight loss. Although it differs dramatically in meaning, I still consider this f-word to very much be a "curse word" when used to describe a weight problem. I'm referring here to the "f-word" *fat*. Whenever you use this particular f-word regarding your body image, you are obviously judging yourself in a belittling manner. That's because the word "fat" invokes images—consciously or unconsciously—of another

weight-loss curse word, which I label the "u-word"—
ugly. Unfortunately, the combination of the f-word plus
the u-word can unleash your IB on you, with self-sabotaging consequences regarding your weight-loss efforts virtually guaranteed.

To understand this concept better, follow the conversation below, which all too typically repeats in many
households.

Kristy has an appealing but slightly chunky body,
which is nonetheless the envy of some of her friends.
Kristy is dressing for a dinner party, which she and her
husband Roger will attend. The following dialogue
ensues:

Kristy: (with distress in her voice) "How do I look?
Do I look fat?"

Roger: (with a tinge of annoyance because he
has heard the question so often over many
years) "Absolutely not. You look great in
that outfit."

Kristy: "Do you really mean that?"

Roger: "Of course I do."

Kristy: "Honest? I don't believe you. You're just
saying that so I don't get upset before the
party."

What you as an observer can't know is that a second "conversation" is taking place simultaneously, un-
heard by Roger. This is mainly an internal exchange
within Kristy's mind, and it too is triggered by the judgmental quality inherent in the word fat.

Kristy: (to herself) "I feel fat."

IB:　 "You are fat! And as a result, you're pretty ugly too...undesirable and unlovable to boot!"

Kristy: "Oh, my gosh; if that's true, Roger will probably end up leaving me or maybe cheat on me. How can I be sure he really believes I'm not too fat?"

IB:　 "Go ahead and ask him." (she does)

Kristy: "He says I'm not fat."

IB:　 "Oh, stop. You know you don't believe him for one second. You've got to trust me and not him, just like you always do at times like this!"

A Two-Edged Sword

Do you see how your negative perception of your body, often exaggerated in your mind, sparks two conversations? These external and internal dialogues are intimately connected. Both are the result of the negative judgment evoked by use of the f-word fat. As underscored above, the word conjures images of "ugliness," which in turn can leave you feeling deep down as though you are basically worthless, if not outright unlovable. This, in turn, represents the type of harsh, if not cruel, self-judgment that your IB would love you to believe about yourself—permanently.

Suppose you stand on the scale, after a joyous holiday season of wining and dining, and discover you added ten pounds or gained enough to increase two clothing sizes. In reality, although you have become just a bit overweight, chances are your perception of yourself will be that you are now *fat*. Even if you are, in fact, significantly overweight, there is no rational reason to judge yourself using this f-word—and in the process energize your IB against you. Let me recommend you instead only use words like "large-framed," "Rubenesque," or even"voluptuous" in characterizing your body image. While these words do suggest that you are well beyond your normal height/weight balance, they are nowhere as judgmental as the word fat. They won't automatically lead you to view yourself at the core as ugly. Hopefully, they will spur you to action and help you avoid any lapse in your efforts to shed those excess pounds.

The f-word is like a two-edged sword, with one edge sharper and more damaging than the other. It can discourage, if not destroy, a person's determination to lose weight, and thus create a sense of vulnerability and resignation. If this is the case, any commitment to a diet and exercise program is likely to be undermined, sooner or later—the door is opened and the "welcome mat" is rolled out, inviting further sabotaging by your IB.

As a little aside, although its negative connotation almost always predominates, the word *fat*, on occasion, can have a positive influence. For a limited number of people, it can serve as a motivator to lose weight. In these instances, the f-word creates enough shame and embarrassment so that your vow to lose weight and never stray from your efforts is actually upheld over the long haul.

The "S-Word"

When you think about losing weight and keeping it off, you often project into the future and imagine having a sleek and toned body—indeed, a "skinny" body. It may surprise you to know that using this word, or its virtual synonym "thin," can in my view be every bit as harmful to reaching your weight-loss goal as the use of the f-word fat.

Our society today is "skinny-driven." Magazines, newspapers, and television repeatedly reiterate the message that being skinny/thin is "in!" Each time you thumb through a magazine or newspaper or watch television, the message is pounded home: skinny, skinny, skinny. Fashions are presented on bony-thin bodies in each fashion journal. Skinny/thin has become the ideal—in stark contrast to periods in the past when society expected/wanted women to be shapely, if not ample. From teenagers to seniors, women of all ages dream of emulating these gaunt models of today. Yet pursuing a skinny/thin body is the equivalent of the pursuit of "perfection"—which, as previously underscored, is perfectly impossible to attain! That is exactly why I have designated the word *skinny* as another weight-loss curse word, which combined with the f-word covers both extremes of the body-image—and, therefore, the judgmental—spectrum.

A Dangerous Route

Far too many girls and younger women (not just gender related—10 percent of anorexics are male) fantasize over extreme sculpted bodies. You've heard the comment, "That's a body to kill for." Unfortunately, they can in fact be killers, but in a very dissimilar way. Many professional models suffer from serious eating disorders like anorexia, bulimia, or some form of both. The first is characterized by an obsession to become excessively thin through excessive diet (i.e., restricting); the second is characterized by episodes of secretive binge eating followed by self-induced vomiting (i.e., purging).

Either of these disorders can be quite hazardous to your health as you strive to emulate a model's "twiggy-like" body. If you were intent on becoming a professional model, the agony might be worthwhile because of the high wages top models earn. But for the average person, this is a goal far too dangerous and too difficult to reach, and is the kind of unrealistic, self-sabotaging challenge on which your Bully thrives.

Deep inside, your IB knows the goal of being—and staying—skinny/thin is unachievable for almost everyone. The conflict manifests itself in constant attempts to slim down, without success. As you struggle for an unrealistic result, the Bully knows you will eventually stop and manufacture excuses to end or delay your efforts. Worse, it may diabolically tempt you to focus on the s-word until, sooner or later, you become ill, by falling into the quagmire of anorexia or bulimia. So be forewarned: if and when your IB ever urges you to reduce your food intake significantly, stop and take notice. This signals that the Bully intends to sabotage your weight-loss struggle by pushing you toward an unobtainable target that guarantees only that you will stumble and fail miserably.

Absolutes versus Comparatives

Some years ago, while conducting a therapy session, something occurred to me for the first time. My patient, Sasha, was venting over her never-ending frustration about losing weight and keeping it off. She suddenly blurted out a statement that initially sounded rather unremarkable to me. Upon further consideration though, I realized this statement was a breakthrough of sorts. Specifically, Sasha stated, "I'd be thrilled just to be skinnier, even if that meant I wasn't truly skinny."

Skinny is an absolute term; whereas skinn<u>ier</u> is a relative term. At that moment, I realized the simplicity and, at the same time, significance of Sasha's statement. Absolutes are often impossible standards to achieve. The pursuit of "perfect"—in this case a model's skinny/thin body—means that you likely have set a magical number you consider necessary to reach to be skinny. The number may be in pounds or in clothing size. Whatever that number is for you, reaching any level short of it will most likely feel at best disappointing, and at worst shattering. It will probably cause you to quit and once again seek comfort from the fridge or pantry.

Consider Sasha as you pursue your weight-loss goal. Promise yourself to eliminate the words fat or skinny when thinking or talking about your body image. It's okay to think of yourself as "heavier" than you'd like to be, but not fat. When you adopt a plan to reduce your weight, make certain it involves becoming skin<u>nier</u> or thin<u>ner</u>, and not skinny or thin. Aim to reach a *range* of pounds, rather than a specific number of pounds (or clothing size), allowing you the flexibility to feel a solid accomplishment even if you "only" attain the upper end of the range.

Descriptive Words Can Help

As you continue to ascertain weight-loss plans, you might consider adding a descriptive word or two to your goal. When doing this, your actual size will determine the most appropriate term. For example, you may be a "little bit" heavy or even "significantly" overweight— clearly more gentle terms are more descriptive of your reality than simply the word fat. On the other end of the weight spectrum, you may attempt to become a "little bit" slimmer, "moderately" more slender, or "significantly" skinnier/thinner. All of these preferable descriptive terms can exert a positive influence on how you evaluate your external self.

In closing, let me once again encourage you to be much more mindful than you likely ever have been regarding the virtually universal curse words of weight-loss efforts: fat and skinny/thin. By being more aware of the ultimately self-sabotaging effects of these words on you, you will eventually be able to counter the curse (and thus the curse <u>words</u>) of your IB—and eventually progress along your weight-loss path.

Now we move to the next Block: loyalty issues.

Chapter 8
INNER BLOCK NUMBER FOUR:
LOYALTY ISSUES

* * *

Think back to your childhood days. Picture your parents as they were when you were growing up. How were they built? Were they moderately heavy, or significantly overweight? How about your siblings? And what about you?

Focus in next on the role food played in your family's lifestyle. Was eating an important part of the family agenda? Was the daily menu chock full of sugars, or starches, or outright fattening foods? Did you, for example, have a robust Italian momma stressing, "Mangia, mangia"? Or perhaps a Jewish mother urging you to, "Es, mein kind"? How many times did you hear, "Finish everything," or "Clean your plate"? Did your folks lay a guilt trip on you with the admonition, "Think of all the starving kids in Africa"?

I have just two more questions and then I'm done. When you think of the role food and eating played in the family before you left the old homestead, was eating together a pleasant experience? Was the emphasis placed on stuffing yourself, or on eating healthy foods with healthy limits? Your responses to all these questions will tell you a great deal about the impact your childhood involvement with food has had on your current weight problems—and on how difficult it is to break away from those family customs.

Disloyalty at the Dinner Table

Not too long ago, Donald, who is a very determined weight-loss patient, visited my office. He had just traveled several hundred miles to spend a weekend at his parents' home celebrating a dear cousin's fiftieth birthday. He was chagrined by the experience. He hadn't seen his family in some time, and encountered his mom to be the chunky, warm, loving lady who still, to this day, seemed to thrive on her ampleness. His dad, who was always a bit overweight, clearly had gained some hefty poundage himself. Donald's siblings were a good deal heavier than when he had last seen them. They apparently had not made the effort he had to trim off those unwanted rolls of fat. In striking contrast, Donald had slimmed down over the past few months, because he was meticulous in following the eating program his nutritionist had devised for him, which then was reinforced during his sessions with me.

Before they had even sat down for the first dinner of the weekend, Donald found himself chided with comments by some of the others—"You look too thin," "Are you feeling okay?" Then it was time to gather around mom's table, as the extended family had for years, and savor the goodies that made her the "tribe's" culinary star. An invitation to one of mom's meals was a prized event. Nonetheless, Donald was determined to adhere as closely as he could to his diet. In fact, he had telephoned a day or so before his arrival to let "Chef Mom" know that he was on a diet and determined to continue eating in a healthy way.

While everyone around him gobbled up the fatty, carb-crammed, sugar-glutted dishes that came out one after the other, Donald treated them as a nothing more than a mini tasting-menu, taking just a bit from each. With each serving came another instruction to eat, "Have more. It's delicious!" When Donald resisted, he was told, "Come on. It's okay to indulge once in a while for goodness sake!" Or worse yet, "You're hurting Momma by not eating. It's an insult 'cause you know how good her food is."

Donald began to waver as this obvious guilt-tripping intensified. He couldn't face his mother's sad look as she asked, "What's the matter? You don't like my cooking anymore?" He finally caved completely when his dad chimed in with, "Momma looked forward so much to your coming home. What's happened to you? Why can't you be like all the rest of us here and just enjoy yourself?" Needless to say, when Donald finally arrived at my office for his next session, he was still reeling from the conflicting pressures of his loyalty and love for his family, versus his determination to lose weight.

Bonding and Loyalty

I would hope that the emotional connection you feel with your family is based on a great deal more than just the enjoyment of sharing festive meals together. Nevertheless, being overweight and/or overindulgent with food like the rest of your immediate family just might be one of the ties bonding you together. Certainly, you may feel a strong kinship, a love, indeed a loyalty, to your family that extends far beyond considerations of body size. But for some people, at least on a subconscious level anyway, a family-related, food-oriented attachment is quite powerful. In fact, you might think of the following simple equation as being the essence of the circumstances: overeating plus being overweight equals an act of loyalty across overweight family members!

Most people think of loyalty in purely positive terms, that is, a relationship that benefits both parties. Yet loyalty, at times, can be detrimental, particularly when either person is harmed by his/her dedication to the bond. It is much like the marital bond—"for better or for worse." When a mate has been found cheating, the unhappy spouse should not necessarily be expected to remain loyal to that vow. That's equally true when a family member who is dedicated to shedding pounds feels a deep sense of loyalty to the family's heritage of obesity.

Of course, it is quite unlikely that family members who are overweight themselves will ever directly admonish you for disloyalty. But that doesn't really matter, because their expectations of loyalty are voiced in their (again) guilt-inducing comments like, "You look too thin" or "Are you trying to take off weight?" In truth, they are indirectly protesting that you have abandoned the dinner-table "glue" that bonds the family together— and that you, therefore, should feel guilty as a result.

Perhaps not on a conscious level, but certainly you should feel guilt on a subconscious level—that's the basic underlying message here.

But here's where your ever-present IB surfaces once again. The IB knows that you care deeply about your parents, siblings, and probably other family members too. It is very much aware that feelings of loyalty and love for these people may be extremely important to you. It counts on the likelihood that when you eat in a controlled manner and manage your weight properly, you will get a misleading reaction from some of these loved ones who don't want to hurt you, yet may feel deep down that you have "abandoned" them.

Instead of condemning your alleged disloyalty, they may flatter you by saying things like, "Gosh you looked so great before, but I guess you still look good now too," or "Ummm, I guess a congratulations for sticking with it is in order." Watch their body language and their facial expressions carefully. You will often discover that they mean quite the opposite. It is their subtle way of sending you a message of resentment because you have chosen to be different and have been so successful at it. If not on the surface, then deep in the recesses of your mind you begin to sense that they have camouflaged their true feelings in supportive phrases that trigger your guilt and summon your IB to action.

Enmeshment

You may be wondering whether this kind of subconscious loyalty to being overweight is common. In my lengthy professional experience, the best answer is yes, but primarily in what are known as "enmeshed families." These are families which are overly close-knit. The members are so attached to one another that they do a relatively poor job of setting boundaries. Most everyone automatically shares each member's stress or pain. Because of this excessive closeness, the success of one member can occasionally foster a feeling of "desertion"—disloyalty—on the part of the others.

Let's apply that principle to weight loss. If you are successful in your efforts to lose weight and keep it off, at least one or more of your enmeshed loved ones may feel (again) deserted, and possibly even jealous of your success. Whatever their motivation, you will begin to sense their resentment. That, in turn, will open the door to feelings of disloyalty and guilt on your part. At that point, in steps the Bully. It takes over inside you, and reinforces those sentiments. If you then allow those negative feelings to become intense enough, that guilt, boosted by your IB, will bring you "back into the fold" as a loyal family member. As a result, you will end up eating far too much, and chances are you eventually will regain all that weight you struggled so hard to lose. That almost happened to Donald, the case study I described earlier in this chapter. Fortunately, it took only two relapse-prevention sessions to put him back on his success track.

Switching Loyalties

The challenge you face is the very fundamental need to shift your underlying sense of loyalty from your family members to <u>yourself</u>, on matters of healthy eating (as well as exercising). This does not mean abandoning them. You and each member of your family can still share healthy loyalties. For example, you can laugh together at joyous moments or cry together over misfortunes. You can continue to love all of them with all of your heart and soul and participate actively in all but one aspect of their routine—you cannot eat uncontrollably as they often enough do.

The key to finding the most suitable balance to help you overcome the loyalty Block lies therefore in *guilt management*. You must face up to the fact that your enmeshment-related guilt is steering you into an ambush. You are being pressured—more by yourself than by others, but with the prodding of your IB—to forsake all that you have worked so hard to achieve on the weight-loss front. Your misguided loyalty to your family is morphing into loyalty to overeating, which guarantees only that you will return to overweight status, much like the rest of your relatives.

That choice should not be so hard to make. As I pointed out above, you can continue to be a loyal and devoted family member on many levels, despite your commitment to attaining a healthy weight and an attractive body. But if you lose your self-esteem because you have capitulated to what you experience inside as a loyalty issue, the ramifications will be felt in all aspects of your life.

Never forget that losing weight is an act of loyalty to the person who always should be your number-one priority—you of course! In reality, it does no harm to those loved ones who do not have the same degree of inner fortitude or courage to stick to their convictions as you do. Share your heart and your soul with them, as I said earlier, but realize that you owe them nothing when you refuse to join in their all-too-many episodes of overindulgent eating.

On now to the next Block to losing weight—emotional overeating.

Chapter 9
INNER BLOCK NUMBER FIVE:
EMOTIONAL OVEREATING

* * *

Try this short exercise to introduce the next proposed IBL to losing weight. Just fill in the blank to
the following sentence. Feel free to enter more than
one answer; several answers are common for most
people.

"In all honesty, I tend to eat more than I should
or things that I shouldn't especially when I am feeling _____." In my experience presenting
this question to people, the most common responses
given are bored, sad, angry, anxious, disappointed,
jealous, stressed, and exhausted. Oh, and certainly
unresolved, lingering *guilt* is on this list—whether in regard to something you recently did that you really can't
forgive yourself for, or even something in your distant
past. Actually, taking guilt as a trigger for overeating
one more step, how about this for a paradox: sometimes you may feel guilty enough about straying from
your diet that you end up choosing, consciously or
subconsciously, to overeat even more, as though you
are feeling so guilty inside that you basically *punish*

yourself by more uncontrolled eating! I'll just leave this idea about guilt as food for thought for you. This list of possible emotional triggers for uncontrolled eating does not exhaust all the possibilities—so don't hesitate to come up with some of your own choices not on the list.

Just as a mostly negative or unhappy state of mind can trigger a craving for food, so can the absence of positive emotions. A feeling that the pleasurable things in life are passing you by and/or that your life is sometimes, if not often, hollow and unfulfilled can add up to you likely feeling emotionally *deprived*. As a result, you can turn to food to fill a "pleasure void" in your life. Or, more specifically, you might overeat, perhaps to soothe a "companionship void," or possibly a "sexual void." In each of these cases, you may end up turning to your most loyal and ardent "friends" to fill that sense of emptiness, that is, your fridge and your pantry.

Suppressing Negative Emotions

Let's take a look at Jeff, a resistant patient who required a good deal of therapy before we were able to resolve his underlying issues. Jeff was moody and whiney, caused especially by his unhappiness over working in the family's retail furniture business. Jeff wanted to be a musician, but his musical skills weren't of a quality that could financially support him and his expanding family. So Jeff reluctantly left the music world and agreed to join the family business. While he always had a husky build, with a tendency toward being overweight, once Jeff started working at the store those pounds began to multiply noticeably.

Amazingly, Jeff claimed he hardly ever experienced any negative emotions of any type. He also insisted to me that he didn't see himself as being moody or a "downer" of a person. That's because, over the years, Jeff had developed a very specific and consistent way of dealing with depressing and/or anxiety-producing moments when they rose to the surface. Simply speaking, he ate! Yes, Jeff basically suppressed or "squelched" his negative, upsetting feelings far down inside him-self—especially with chips, hoagies, or buttery popcorn. In fact, he had mastered this "squelching" technique so well that it became reflexive, to the glee of his approving IB. With therapy, however, Jeff learned to express negative feelings to others in a more open and direct way, rather than revert back to his life-long pattern of squelching these emotions through overeating.

Dealing With Emotions of Deprivation

You recall that I mentioned that the absence of *positive* emotions could also cause you to eat emotionally. Your sense of deprivation, of missing out on the more enjoyable and rewarding aspects of life, can start you toward the fridge for solace. My patient Faye knew that only too well.

Faye worked on the assembly line at a local manu-facturing plant. It was not a very rewarding occupa-tion, but Faye found it hard to obtain a better job since she had dropped out of high school before earning a diploma. An unpleasant divorce from James added to her sense of deprivation. She had few friends to turn to, but she was not a socially comfortable woman. She felt lonely and lacking in any real accomplishment in her life, and was a classic example of an emotional eater when she arrived in my office.

Faye explained that she felt entitled to at least some pleasures in her dull life, and eating without restrictions was at the top of the list. She worked all day on her shift at the plant, came home to an empty house, and headed straight to the kitchen for comfort. Faye's simple "pleasure principle" required no social effort on her part. She needed no other person to interact with her. She found it a very easy relationship to maintain. But this simple pleasure principle had, of course, an equally simple downside. Faye became larger and larger and, therefore, less appealing to men and even to potential women friends as she continued to gorge day after day.

It took us a bit of time to untangle all of the conflicting forces in Faye's past that brought her to this self-demeaning situation. Most important was to make her realize, in contrast to her Bully's harangues, that food was not the panacea for the many problems she faced. She had to be made to understand that yes, she was suffering from deprivation, but it was she and no one else who was the cause. By quitting school, she deprived herself of a complete high school education and the possibility of a more interesting and lucrative career. Her divorce from James and her inability to make and keep friends were very much due to her dour outlook on life. She was suffering from an absence of positive emotional experiences. When Faye finally gained the strength to admit to herself that it was she who created every void in her existence, she was well on the way to restructuring her lifestyle in a positive and productive way.

That realization gave Faye the courage to face down her IB, and accept the fact that the more she turned to uncontrolled eating, the more damage she was doing to herself. She was paying dearly for those brief self-pacifying moments at the fridge by sabotaging any remnant of her weight-loss hopes and shattering her self-esteem, to say nothing of her battered self-image.

There is no question that there are times when everyone—you, me, and the rest of the world—feels a need for comfort and nurturance. Some of us are lucky enough to have someone immediately available to whom we can turn to meet our needs. A hug from someone who cares, and someone willing to listen to us in those depressed moments is far more effective and far less self-defeating than raiding the fridge or pantry.

Resolving "Emotional Eating" Blocks

At the risk of sounding glib or oversimplifying the issue, I assume that you logically are aware that other options are available to you to ease your unhappiness temporarily, aside from overindulgent eating. However, those alternatives are not easy to pursue when food is so conveniently close by—not to mention when your IB is goading you to choose that all-too-easy remedy. Options that can be particularly helpful in dealing with strong negative emotions include emotionally venting to a friend, writing about these emotions in a journal, or something quite soothing like taking a warm bath. Or try channeling your frustrations into a more constructive or distracting activity, like reading, listening to music, or enjoying working on a hands-on project. You may even find that some sexual self-stimulation can be quite helpful, assuming you are comfortable with that.

The key is to find an alternative to distract you from feeling sorry for yourself and consequently allowing your IB to take over. If you choose not to follow any of the diversionary strategies like those listed above, you surrender to the Bully and allow it to steer you directly into the uncontrolled emotional eating that you know you should avoid. Thus you become that much more vulnerable to, shall we say, carb-surrender or sugar-surrender or fatty-food-surrender. Across any of these, the bottom line Across any of these, the bottom line is that you, once again, have given in to the sabotaging efforts of your seductive Bully.

In closing this chapter, my question to you is this: "When you are feeling either emotionally 'down' and/ or that you are missing out on positive or 'up' feelings, will you continue to focus on and give in to the temptation to eat, if not overeat? Or will you opt for a more constructive route to cope with your distressing emotions—and in the process, return to your weight-loss aspirations?" The choice of course is yours, and hopefully your choice will be the wise one!

OK, on to the next possible Block to losing weight—spite.

Chapter 10
INNER BLOCK NUMBER SIX: SPITE

* * *

Joe and Jenna, married for twelve years and counting, were the dictionary definition of the "Bickersons." They squabbled day after day, over a variety of never-ending issues. Their individual litanies of complaints, repeated constantly, were always met with counter-complaints.

As tempers escalated, each partner became increasingly determined to win the battle. Neither ever won nor lost, but their marriage came very close to becoming the ultimate loser. Typically, these exchanges were power struggles that took the form of threats and counter-threats. They were spiteful challenges by two frustrated and hurt people who refused to agree (even when they recognized that their partner possibly might be right). For example:

Jenna: "Joe, you promised faithfully that you'd ask for a raise—so why haven't you done it yet?

Joe: "I told you Jen, first you've got to slim down enough to fit into the new clothes that raise would pay for."

And as the inimitable Kurt Vonnegut used to put it in many of his books, "And so it goes." While Jenna's weight was the trigger for their most frequent and contentious arguments, the couple often squabbled over many other issues too. Often enough, these were relatively petty issues, like a repair to the front porch. So Jenna, for example, would demand that Joe tackle the job and finish it. But then Joe typically responded, "You said you'd clean up the mess in the bedroom closet. I'll do the porch when that happens." At other times, they battled over anything and everything from visiting Jenna's mother, to the frequency of sexual relations, to going out for a special dinner, or a night at the movies.

The "YCF Syndrome"

Once, in the midst of a typical squabble-filled therapy session with Jenna and Joe, Jenna suddenly blurted out, "I'll change, but only when you change first!" I was encouraged that the advice I had repeated at each of their previous sessions might finally be sinking in for this couple. At the very least, Jenna now seemed to recognize they were playing the destructive game of "You change first...no, you first." Once again I explained to the two of them, as I had week after week, that all of this arguing and the insistence that the other partner change first was nothing more than a power struggle. "Each of you refuses to give in to the other's request without demanding something in return," I felt compelled to add.

Thinking about the session later that evening, a light bulb flashed in my mind. I was reminded that these types of power struggles were a problem common to most couples in therapy—and enough couples that never come in for therapy. Common enough for me to coin the descriptive acronym "YCFS," which stands for "You Change First! Syndrome."

The YCFS frequently occurs when one partner in a relationship suffers from obesity, as Jenna did. "You're too fat. Why don't you take those pounds off? You'd look a lot better, and I could be attracted to you again," the Joe's of this world all too often convey to the overweight Jenna's of the world. But then the latter's response inevitably is something like, "I'll slim down when *you* treat me the way I should be treated, with caring and respect!" Of course, this quid pro quo can be over anything more specific. But the essence of these exchanges is pure YCFS—"I'll probably do what you want me to, but only if you do what I want you to do <u>first</u>!"

"Newton's Third Law" Applied

Sometime in the months after I began using the term YCFS with many of my other power-struggling couples, I became intrigued by the similarity between the YCFS and the Third Law of Sir Isaac Newton. As you may recall from your school days, Sir Isaac many moons ago proposed the notion that every action produces an equal and opposite reaction.

Let's now apply that basic notion to the sparring couple we have talked about. Once again, Jenna stated, "I'll change when you change first." That almost always guaranteed an equal and opposite response from Joe of, "No, I'll change when you change first!" It thus appears from this exchange that Sir Isaac could well have been one astute relationship therapist if he hadn't chosen to concentrate on physics!

When YCFS Turns to Spite

You can be certain that your ever-present IB plays a key role in these contentious exchanges, urging each partner to continue down his/her destructive path. Let's expand a little further on the way in which the YCFS and your IB impact relationships in which one partner is overweight. The slimmer partner, for example, may challenge his/her mate along the lines of, "When you finally take off weight, we can socialize more because I won't be ashamed to be seen with you." With trigger now pulled so to speak, the battle begins, as the overweight mate retorts, "That's just an excuse. Show me you mean it, and I will trim down!" Once again it's "you change first," with your IB applauding in the background. That exchange can be applied to any number of issues. It can be as simple as, "I'll help more around the house if you lose weight." Or perhaps, "I'll make vacation plans when you slim down," or "You'll be a lot more appealing so we can enjoy more sex together." The danger is that the conflict often escalates and includes belittling remarks that range from the relatively mild, "You can't even fit into your clothes anymore," to the vicious, "You're nothing more than a fat pig!"

As you might expect, this level of nastiness can gradually create the impulse toward *spite*. The overweight yet maligned partner feels extremely resentful. That resentment, in turn, may intensify over time, and lead to a desire to spite the maligning partner—once again urged on by the Bully. This may not occur on a conscious level, but it certainly can exist subconsciously. In either case, these spiteful impulses become a powerful IBL to losing weight for the Jennas of the world who are coupled off with the Joes of the world.

I recall a statement that Jenna made at one of our sessions that demonstrates this concept so well. "Joe makes me so mad with his threats and belittling comments that at times I refuse to continue with my weight-loss program just to piss him off!" So you can see how Jenna spites Joe for his insensitive, hurtful comments.

Unfortunately, Jenna isn't spiting just her husband. Let's face it: she becomes a victim of her spite herself! Look at the dynamic that's involved. Jenna, in essence, chose a trade-off. In her effort to aggravate and spite Joe, she undermined her own efforts to reduce her weight. A poor trade-off perhaps, but Jenna had reached the point of feeling so insulted and exasperated by Joe's offensive comments that she was willing to sabotage herself in order to spite him. As she told me, "You reach a point where you decide you will not be passive and give in to his threats and insults any longer!"

Tackling the Spite Block

The key to controlling the "spite Block" is to determine your <u>priorities</u>. That is, you owe it to yourself to undertake actions in the order of their importance to you, rather than allowing your emotions or the urgings of your IB to control you. So even if you feel justified in allowing your anger at the callous remarks of your partner to hurt him/her back, you must first consider the harm it will do to *you*. After all, you are fully aware that losing weight is your priority. You know that you, therefore, must resist the urge to spite your partner, because you will only damage yourself. So you must act accordingly and control yourself!

When you find yourself in situations like this, always remember that your weight loss comes first. Even if you feel that you would be "giving in" by not responding spitefully, realize that losing weight benefits you far more than it does your partner. Don't sacrifice your own welfare just for the momentary satisfaction of upsetting him/her. Remind yourself every day, "I will lose weight and keep it off for <u>my own</u> sake, no matter what comments I may get from him/her. I want to look and feel attractive for my own benefit. I refuse to keep sacrificing my self-esteem and my self-respect!"

Your ability to control the impulse to spite won't happen overnight. But you will see improvement just as soon as you begin to moderate your anger by recognizing the damage you do to yourself when you abandon your weight-loss goal just to spite your partner. Give yourself three to six months to stay on this mental track. The drive to spite has likely been in-grained in your conscious or subconscious mind for a good amount of time. If you persist in your efforts to prioritize losing weight, however, you will find that, over time, you will be able to control your urge to spite—whether your relationship with your partner improves, remains the same, or becomes worse.

Chapter 11
THE "TEN COMMANDMENTS" OF SUCCESSFUL WEIGHT LOSS

* * *

Preface: In Sum...........

So there you have it. You now understand the ways in which your IB continually attempts to undermine your every effort to shed excess pounds. We spent a good deal of time together in this book examining the six primary psychological obstacles to weight loss that I refer to as Inner Blocks. It should now be clear that your Inner Bully could use any IBLs as the culprit or culprits sabotaging your efforts to lose weight and keep it off.

We started our review of the six primary IBLs by analyzing the most universal and troublesome one—addiction to self-rebellion. With that as an introduction to the way the Blocks work, we moved on to the various forms of approach-avoidance tendencies that an anxiety Block can cause, then to the judgmental tone of certain body image "curse words." Then we looked at conflicts involving loyalty Blocks that you may feel inside. Next, we focused on how a variety of negative feelings or feeling deprived of pleasure in your life can cause an emotional overeating Block. And we concluded our investigation of the most common IBLs by helping you realize that when the spite Block induces you to retaliate against a significant other by eating uncontrollably, you are really harming yourself much more than your partner/antagonist.

Each of these Blocks is a catalyst for action by your IB. Once it gains a foothold, the Bully will continue its efforts to woo you away from your program of carefully regulated eating and exercising. If you allow it to take control, the Bully will, as you know by now, continue until it achieves total victory—and that of course translates to total defeat for you!

Add to that scenario to the fact that, as underscored in Chapter 1, the mass of diet and exercise programs proliferating today fail when you essentially cede control to the Bully. Their claims of producing the sleek bodies they picture in their ads are obviously misleading when you see the number of participants who fail to achieve weight goals while enrolled in their programs. This, in turn, is a reminder, once again, of the disclaimers cleverly buried in a corner or at the bottom of these ads, stating that results "may vary" or "are not typical."

All of this, let me emphasize, is in no way intended to demean dieting and exercise! On the contrary, from my perspective, the ultimate irony is that you can choose to follow almost any diet and exercise program, and end up successfully losing weight– but only by taking control of your body and overcoming the IBLs affecting you. And the one "Block" that can greatly increase your chances of achieving success is your blocking of: your IB, from sabotaging your efforts to lose weight and keep it off!

Hope Abounds

A little over a year ago, I decided to offer to the public an IB/IBL *treatment program*, for those individuals mired in the struggle to lose weight and keep it off. Three considerations especially motivated me to offer this unique program:

1. As underscored back in Chapter One, the recidivism rate for people who try to lose weight, but end up regaining it is generally accepted to be 90 percent or higher.
2. My recognition of the self-sabotaging role of the IB, and the importance of doing what you can not to let it control you.
3. My firm belief that inner or psychological Blocks to losing weight undermine almost everyone's efforts to lose weight, regardless of the specific diet or exercise program you may be utilizing.

The preliminary success to date of my program led me to write this book, in the hope of introducing the concept to a larger audience. While I am eagerly waiting for outcomes from a greater number of patients, I do feel that the results obtained so far justify introducing the program publicly. Participants vary widely in the number of sessions they have spent in treatment. Some have reached success with a minimal three to five treatment visits, while other have gone well beyond ten sessions. Some participants have completed treatment, while others are still making regular visits to my office. Because of these variables, as well as the relatively small number of patients overall who have been in my program to date, I hesitate to announce any firm conclusions regarding the success of my program.

Nonetheless, I want to share with you some very encouraging preliminary results. Of the ten patients who have attended treatment sessions principally for the purpose of addressing and resolving their IBLs and losing weight, five of those ten have maintained their desired weight for an extended period of time, that is, at least six months. Two of the remaining five are in the three to six month category, and the other three are in the category of too-soon-to-tell.

I am pleased about the 50 percent success rate to date, because it certainly encourages me to continue to offer and build upon my IBLs program. Periodic follow-up assessments have been conducted by myself and my assistant to monitor maintenance of treatment benefits. Most participants readily and enthusiastically respond to these assessments with very positive feedback.

Let me also underscore that the participants in my program have followed a wide variety of different diet programs, including Weight Watchers, the Atkins Diet, NutriSystems, Jenny Craig, and personally-tailored nutrition programs. I think you'll agree that these early positive results from my program indicate that working to control your IB and overcome your particular IBLs can potentially increase your odds of successfully trimming pounds on <u>any</u> diet and exercise program!

I encourage you to participate in your own anti-Bully/ anti-Blocks program. When you accept the challenge and follow the regimen I have prescribed in this book, I hope you will be kind enough to contact me, either in person, by telephone, or by e-mail, so your results can be validated and added to the growing body of positive outcomes. That way, other practitioners, and the millions of Americans who are facing weight problems, can all then benefit from your hopefully gratifying experience.

The "Ten Commandments" of Weight Loss

Before closing this book, I want to leave you with some guidelines—"commandments" if you will—to refer to any time you feel discouraged by the slow progress of your weight loss. These "commandments" have absolutely no relationship of course to anything religious. They mainly are a set of recommendations, to guide you in your daily efforts to control your IB and surmount any IBLs to losing weight that you may up against. Here they are, in the form of "You will" statements rather than in the original religious "Thou shall" wording:

1. You will make no vows or resolutions about losing weight that you do not fully intend to keep.
2. You will recognize your IB as being your self-sabotaging "inner enemy," and proceed to create a symbolic object for your IB to help you fight back and control it better.

3. You will make a list of your IBLs and commit yourself to resolving those that have been sabotaging you.

4. You will work on controlling your "addiction to self-rebellion" Block—especially in terms of being a responsible adult who maintains self-discipline on the eating and exercising fronts.

5. You will virtually chant the following *mantra* to yourself several times a day, especially prior to any meal or snack: "Self-control means self-respect and self-esteem!"

6. You will remind yourself every day that your true self-esteem depends more on what you like about yourself on the *inside* than on looking good on the outside.

7. You will weigh yourself as <u>infrequently</u> as possible while trying to lose weight.

8. You will give yourself some credit at day's end every time you have a "good day" of controlling your eating and getting some exercise.

9. You will give yourself the desirable option of consulting with your family doctor or nutritionist to design a healthy-eating program, and a personal trainer to help you with the best type of exercise for you.

10. Last but not least, you will contact a psychotherapist to help you control your IB and tackle your IBLs if you find you cannot do this on your own.

Just as we are expected to follow all of the biblical Ten Commandments and not pick and choose, the same rule applies to <u>my</u> so-called ten commandments. If you truly want to lose weight and keep it off, you must uphold every one of them—absolutely none of them can be considered optional!

In closing, when you think about adherence to this list of "You wills," think of each violation as a weight-loss "sin." So make up your mind firmly—no more sinning! Adhere faithfully to your weight-loss program. Then and only then do you stand a real chance of winning the proverbial "battle of the bulge" once and for all!

REFERENCES

1) <u>The Beck Diet Solution</u>—Judith Beck, Ph.D.; Oxmoor House, 2007
2) <u>Shrink Yourself: Break Free From Emotional Eating</u>—Roger Gould, M.D.; John Wiley And Sons, 2007
3) <u>The Ultimate Weight Loss Solution</u>—Phil McGraw, Ph.D.; Free Press, 2003
4) <u>Personality and Psychotherapy</u>—John Dollard, Ph.D and Neal E.Miller, Ph.D.; Mc-Graw Hill, 1963.
5) <u>Eating Disorders: Anorexia and the Person Within</u>—Hilde Bruch, M.D.; Basic Books, 1985
6) <u>Handbook of Personality and Self-Regulation</u>—Jennifer Crocker, Ph.D.; John Wiley and Sons, 2009
7) "A Theory of Human Motivation"—Abraham Maslow; in <u>Psychological Review</u>, 50(4), 1943
8) "How To Curb Your Hunger"—Krista Scott-Dixon, Ph.D.; blog entry

Made in the USA
Charleston, SC
26 February 2010